Love is expressed in routines over time
Love withstands changes

— Author's quote

Peering Through the Keyhole

Peering Through the Keyhole

Janey's Viewpoint

Janey Davies

urlink PRINT & MEDIA

Peering Through the Keyhole

1603 Capitol Ave., Suite 310 Cheyenne, Wyoming USA 82001
1-888-980-6523 | admin@urlinkpublishing.com

URLink Print and Media is committed to excellence in the publishing industry.

Published in the United States of America

Library of Congress Control Number: 2025911916
ISBN 979-8-89690-187-7 (Paperback)
ISBN 979-8-89690-189-1 (Digital)

11.07.25

Table of Contents

Introduction

"When he was a boy, Janey was there when Jimmy learned his first walk." I thought I was his constant, but a wedge has been thrust between us.

Our relationship is in overcast.

An outside-looking in or out-of-the-box insight and experience on family and relationships close to ground zero impacted by with special needs—the struggles, how they were handled, how they were overcome, what matters, and what is reality. Also, a peek at culture touched by modernization or nuance over the span of decades. Jimmy and Janey—other lives maybe harsher, harder, simpler, less eventful than theirs, but it's finite. If you don't live your dreams, you will work to build someone else's.

Chapter 1

Call Out His Name: A Mere Coincidence

"Jimmy, Jimmy!" but the two-year old boy continued running around. This caused grandparents to be concerned since he seems unaware when called by his name. Sometimes, by chance he would turn around, but not all the time. He'd turn to the one calling him as if by mere coincidence. Jimmy is a pale boy with bright eyes and dark hair. He was left under the care of his grandparents, Jonathan and Nancy, while Samantha was away. His older sister, Janey, kept him company in the summers or whenever she was off school. Janey lives with their dad, Mathew, in the city, who also visits Jimmy every chance he gets.

Samantha is smart. She topped the national board, she was away completing her thesis when she had Jimmy. She came home on a school break to be with Janey, her daughter, and Mathew when she became pregnant with Jimmy. Finishing her Masters, she had to leave him with her parents' care for the time being. Matthew had a lot on his plate—his work and attending to Janey. The grandparents happily agreed to the set up.

Samantha was sent to her Masters on a scholarship by her institution. It was a rare and hard opportunity to miss. Jimmy came unexpectedly. Samantha's roommate contracted German measles. She was expecting, too. Sadly, her baby did not survive, so Samantha was thankful to have Jimmy, a healthy baby boy with ten fingers and ten toes. But in the back of her head, she knew it was too good to be true. She is a physician—she knows all too well. Janey, however, four years older than Jimmy was just trying to be like any kid her age and a dutiful older sister as best she can. Janey, unlike Jimmy, was paler. As kids, they normally put on weight in the summers, during school breaks, and turn skinny in the middle of the school year. But no matter how much

Janey ate, she was always skinny. I guess you could blame it on children's metabolism.

Because of those summers, Janey and Jimmy were very close to their grandparents, especially their granddad. They were their spoiled kids. Janey remembers how she could get away with ice cream for breakfast—not always but she could. They never forgot to give them milk, and since Janey just has had it with milk she complained. They'd make her cocoa instead. People at her grandparents' adjusted to her whims *dry smile*

Jimmy since spent most of his toddler years with his grandpa. Samantha's Masters or graduate school studies were finally done and dusted, so she personally came to pick him up. But Jimmy barely knew her, regardless if she visited him every chance she got. There were no cellphones yet so she wrote and wrote and even paid those long distance calls, which were exorbitantly expensive. It was too painful for Samantha that Jimmy barely recognized her. He would hide behind the legs of his grandfather being the two-year old that he is, like his grandpa was his dad or parent.

Samantha made it her mission that "my son will recognize me. By golly! He will answer to me, look up to me, and will want to be with me." She accomplished that. She requested her parents to step back and, almost always and everywhere, she took Jimmy with her. It paid off, and it was all good—for the time being.

As time went, Samantha would steal glances at Jimmy. *My perfect boy! She thought.* But Jimmy doesn't respond when his name was called. They concluded that when he would turn around when called, it was only by chance.

Jimmy was four years old when he was tested, and it was confirmed. He was deaf-mute. Normally, kids would turn around to a clapping sound. He wouldn't. Jimmy responds to a car honking and fireworks. His left ear was a hundred percent deaf, while his right was sixty. He is not totally deaf. The term deaf has evolved over the years to hearing impaired or hearing impairment, and more recently, hard of hearing.

With a hearing aid, Jimmy can use it on the ear that could still hear. This device amplifies sound so that a person with hearing loss could hear sound. Jimmy is a child with special needs. There are thirteen disability categories and the categories have spectrums or degrees—from mildest to most severe.

Samantha prayed, thankful for her boy. But she knew that she will have to do more, or does she? She feels a lot for Jimmy. Everyone in the family does.

Chapter 2

Dengue Fever

Janey often wondered whether all children were difficult to be fed. To this day, she could still hear Jimmy's wails echoing through the corridors. Jimmy was too picky when it comes to food, Janey thought they were almost hopeless on what to feed Jimmy; however, he took a liking to pounded or ground rice, which one uses for rice cakes or pudding.

Janey wasn't sure if it was malnutrition or something that caused Jimmy to catch a very bad fever. Jimmy would cry so hard all the more. Janey worried about her brother. She remembered how concerned they were. His platelet dropped, and they needed it to go up. He had dengue fever or breakbone fever, which is caused by a mosquito bite.

They were rocking him to sleep or consoling him. I don't know if it is harder for children with special needs, but it looked pretty hard then. These are Janey's thoughts.

Some of Janey's memories of Jimmy were mostly at their home or at their grandparents', but she also remembers whenever they were at church or at the mall, Janey would pray so hard hoping her brother would have ESP or mental telepathy. She was very much afraid to lose him in a crowd. But it was the other way around, Matthew, their dad, always had a vivid memory of Jimmy punching another boy at church whom he saw pushed Janey. Ahwwww, so cute, the protective brother.

Jimmy and Janey did many things together. They fought, played, and even celebrated birthdays together. They were both born in January.

They both played superhero together and would tie towels on their necks as capes. They would happily jump up and down their queen-sized bed when…*oops*. That time Janey thought that everything was going alright, she noticed that Jimmy was suddenly gone. He was just right there beside her, jumping by the bed with his own cape, then she found him underneath the cabinet, bleeding. He had fallen, slipped underneath, and hit the edge of the cabinet. They tended to his wound. He looked like a pope—they had to shave the area of the wound. It was white and round on his head, exactly by the hair whorl or cowlick.

They would also take turns in Samantha's sewing machine. She also used to knit, cross-stitch, and all. The machine was made of metal but with the wooden body. Underneath the sewing machine was a device like a wheel. They pretended they were driving. There was a contraption like a lever where a belt connected the machine's spinning wheel to the pedal's spinning wheel that made a sound. That lever was the honk.

Janey picked up Jimmy from swimming and martial arts lessons. The teachers or instructors were never trained for children with special needs, so she wondered how the lessons went.

Janey was Jimmy's babysitter. Well, at least it felt that way to her sometimes. She wasn't just older but also taller, and sometimes, Jimmy would want to play in the streets for whatever reason Janey could not wrap her head around. She was older, but she was a kid, too, and her younger brother with a hearing disability likes the streets. Alarm signs! They got in a fight where Jimmy bit Janey's hand that it bled, and Janey bit his back in vengeance. Both having minor cuts. How could she explain to make Jimmy understand that playing in the streets was dangerous—with the passing cars and all.

And going back dengue fever isn't a measly thing. One of Jimmy and Janey's cousins caught it the second time around. Janey felt that his blood is susceptible to the mosquitoes since he was not really from around here, or someone who doesn't eat much could also be a likely reason, or it's just really the mosquito bite—particularly, the mosquito with white stripes. It's hard to tell mosquitoes apart, but they say the kind that brings dengue are prevalent during the day and with white stripes or white bands on its legs. But what is worse is the anguish when you have it till it's gone—very high fever, stomach pains for some. She recalled their cousin turned a bit too red also for some time till he recovered. Janey did a report on this in class, and she had all the slides since their mom, Samantha, a doctor, conducted a study and really researched on dengue mosquitoes. Other people or friends who had it did not have it as bad as their cousin. But I guess even so was why Jimmy was in so much pain and wailing even more.

Chapter 3

The Games

Jimmy and Janey's grandparents live near the coast. One summer, Janey visited Jimmy. She was left there by their dad, Matthew, and it was also during the time Samantha was finishing her thesis. Many praised Jimmy when he learned how to walk. I guess that's a milestone for children. By coincidence, he learned, near his second birthday. And at his birthday party, he still had wobbly feet—crooked as a crab—as he walked towards their grandfather. But Jimmy's first walk was on the boardwalk near the house of their grandparents. Jimmy and Janey often go there with their sitter. Janey, with one knee bent, stretched her arms as if waiting for a hug, and Jimmy tried his best to go walk towards his older sister. Janey pinned that memory for keeps.

When he was a boy, Janey was there when Jimmy learned his first walk. Janey thought she was going to be his constant.

The family moved to a new home. Janey was heartbroken—more than heartbroken. But she had no say. Her mom was expecting a third child and the building her grandparents owned, run by her mom on the side, was nearby a lot of places. It was near Samantha's and Matthew's work. It was a walk or nearest to Janey's school and even more accessible to Jimmy's school for children with special needs. Rather than checking up on the building and picking up rent from tenants, it was very convenient to move in since it had more than enough room. This isn't where Samantha's parents live—they owned this building with tenants.

In the coast where they live, it is nearby the little private school that they own and ran. Both Samantha's parents were teachers, and they managed to set aside some and put up some businesses, like the school, and they also owned a building far from the coast where Samantha, Matthew, and family moved.

Janey, in secret, cried almost every night as she became attached to her friends in her old neighborhood, and, to this day, are keeping toe to toe. Their clique has been one of her lifelong friends. She was just devastated by the move. But she managed and had new friends at the new neighborhood, and she also had friends in school. Her old neighborhood friends were her play buddies in the summers if she doesn't go to the coast to her grandparents so having something or someone new around took some getting used to.

Jimmy, however, this is where it becomes more interesting, he's a bit older now.

He loves collecting stuff—he had trading cards and pogs or caps. Little boys his age often exchange or barter even bought and sold these, like characters nowadays in computer games or items.

Janey was paying much attention. Their new neighborhood had several buildings compared to the suburbs or house they came from.

Jimmy now enjoyed going around the neighborhood bartering his cards. Janey felt relieved he wouldn't be playing in the streets so much but concern swept over or took its place. What if people took advantage of Jimmy? For Janey, the hardest part for Jimmy was holding back—she knew she could not be there forever. Jimmy must learn for himself, and Janey must learn distance and restraint, give enough room for him.

There was a wall, and Janey was watering the plants, but she could hear children on the other side. Jimmy was learning sign language in school now and that is taught in English. He doesn't really know to speak their dialect or vernacular.

Other kids used to call him *amang*, a colloquial term that means mute, since he couldn't speak like they could. Janey overheard everything, and she was pleased.

Carlson said," Wow! The *amang* has great, expensive cards. Maybe, he'd trade with me." Jimmy used actions to communicate with them. He usually nodded and pointed.

"Let's see. Let's all trade stuff." Todd said. Carlson pointed to one of Jimmy's cards. Janey supposed because she heard Todd say he'd like to trade this other card instead for Jimmy.

Carlson said, "I don't have that I guess that's okay".

Todd said seeing Jimmy's cards, "Wow! The *amang* has this card." Jimmy wanted to barter one of his cards again. Todd said, "I'll barter that."

Janey just wanted to hear that he could say no and that they wouldn't take advantage of him. She was pleased indeed.

Todd lived in the building across the street. He lived only with his grandmother, and his dad visits every now and then. Todd was a fairly goodlooking kid like Jimmy. They both had dark eyebrows, wonderful face features. Todd became Jimmy's first best friend.

Todd used to hang out at Jimmy's and Jimmy at theirs. They played computer games. They used to go together meet up with other neighborhood kids.

In the summer, Todd studied taekwondo, whilst Jimmy did his swimming and karatedo.

***moving ranked top on the stress level list. It's even noted somewhat more stressful than loss in the family—that was on a poll or survey.*

Chapter 4

The Car Accident

Children are resilient, but none as resilient as Jimmy.

There was a knock on the door, and Janey's heart was pounding. For whatever reason, it really did. Maybe because she had an inkling. Minutes before the knock, Janey had gone out the apartment to check that the door to the building had been locked. Jimmy was screeching happily, he was playing with one of the tenants. As long as the door was closed, everything and everyone was safe.

When she opened the door, she saw Jonathan (the same name as their grandfather), a tenant, was carrying Jimmy. Jimmy smiled at Janey, but as soon as his eyes looked at his foot, his face was in disbelief, and he cried. Jonathan hurriedly brought Jimmy to the nearest hospital. Moments later, Samantha arrived home from the compound where the hospital was but from a different building. She was teaching student-doctors or interns. She taught those taking up medicine as she is a doctor or physician. She rushed to the hospital in her high heeled shoes.

Another tenant had gone out and left the door open after Janey had checked. They lived near a school zone—Janey's school—so cars slowed down. But one car, on that fateful day, was in a hurry, heading somewhere else after picking up kids at the school. He was just a driver of a carpool. He accidentally ran over Jimmy's foot the moment he set his foot on the road. The rest of his body still on the sidewalk. No one drove fast there, except that day. Jimmy could not notice as he was hard of hearing and he was playing catch with Andrew, also another tenant. He went straight out of the door as it was open to the street. The worst thing was that the driver drove forward on the foot and when realizing he'd hit someone, upon instinct, backed up—doubly impacting Jimmy's eight-year-old foot.

Jimmy got into a car accident.

As a kid, one of Samantha's sisters wanted to adopt Jimmy. Children with special needs, especially those who are hard of hearing, had more opportunities around her area. It wasn't of an impediment moreso in other places. But Samantha firmly declined; she was a doctor. She can very well take care of her son and, in this car accident, she proved herself beyond a doubt.

Janey, although young, was amazed at how their mother carried the situation.

This was Jimmy's first operation. they took the broken bones out his foot. They were on the verge of amputating his foot. But Samantha put her foot down. When she shared this experience, she remembered thinking, *How terrible it is for my boy to be hard of hearing and have no foot?!*

No.

Jimmy underwent two more operations. They could not perform successive operations in a month. It was that way at that time, some decades ago. Or, maybe, an eight-year old boy was just too fragile. Jimmy was in the hospital for three months. Taking the bone out of the foot was his first operation. His second: skin grafting. They took flesh from his legs instead of from the buttocks since males' buttocks were not that large. They took three bacon-sized, 2-by-5-inch flesh from his legs to graft on his foot that got ran over. They reconstructed his foot for functionality at best.

Jimmy had several tests. Janey was wide-eyed at how Jimmy used to cry whenever a needle was poked on him, but and as the months came along, he'd, ultimately, just extend his arm, as if being injected was normal and an everyday occurrence.

That was the last operation before observation for healing after the skin grafting. He then underwent bone graft for the third. Bone from the hips grew back or regenerate when cut, so they cut a small bone to put on his crushed foot, replacing the broken bones that were removed during the first operation as best they can.

Many things are unimaginable and this is one of them. Photos were essential for the court hearing and the settlement of the car accident. Since Jimmy was hard of hearing and a minor, the plaintiff assumed partial amount in settlement. The family pitched in. Ideally, most only knew amputation at that time and thought that; however, to rescue his foot or for him to be more normally functioning, he underwent a series of more operations. They were all well worth it, just somehow much more out of pocket or costly. It was a school zone, drivers shouldn't rush or overspeed, which was what happened, unfortunately. Since everything could not be covered by the driver, the family stepped in.

Jimmy made it through. He was behind in school, and he missed too much to go back. But one day, after everything, he came home in crutches, and Todd was there.

He easily coped, too.

Children are very resilient. It did not take him long to lose the crutches. A limp isn't even visible. Although, he had bacon scars on his legs and a cut or scar by his hips and a foot reconstructed, which looked like burned flesh was sown onto you, but all five toes were intact. More importantly, he could walk like you and me. Amazing recovery!

Every day, Janey and her family visited Jimmy at the hospital, seeing he had four to five wires supporting his injured foot with wood on both sides. His foot looked like a barbecue, but that was over. All those were removed, and he is fine.

His foot was like on barbecue sticks but using wires as I recall. Janey wondered how this whole ordeal impacted him fully—besides the physical, the psycho-social, and all that. But that was just overthinking; it was a moment of celebration.

Chapter 5

Movies and Bars

Auntie Julie visited one day, and she told Janey "a funny thing" as she called it, even before she told details. She said she walked behind two teenagers along the college where Jimmy's girlfriend studied. The teenagers were giggling saying that there is that handsome boy again we often pass by, picking up his girlfriend from this school. When Auntie Julie turned her head to look at the boy they were referring to, *Oh! That's my nephew,* she thought. They waved— Jimmy and Auntie Julie.

Jimmy was very charming as a kid. He was friendlier than Janey. Janey was a bit reserved and just happy hanging around her crowd.

Jimmy waved, smiled to people, especially whose faces he knew are friends of Samantha, Matthew, or his grandparents. He was never shy.

They sometimes had cousins from Canada visit, and they would go to bars. Jimmy danced. Imagine dancing and you can't hear the beat. Jimmy was cool that way. Jimmy even plays the stereo—says he just pays attention to the vibration, the speakers banging, and the wooden floor slightly moving at home. Well, he explains in sign language. He used to pick up the home phone or landline phone pretending he heard it ring, either it's his jokes or insecurities. At the bar, random girls would come up to him, and he'd have a perplexed face with them talking and asking him to dance, or they'd ask his name. Janey often approached and says he does sign language. He danced better than most; I bet he can fool you. He isn't wonky or anything, not awkward or like that. He is just a regular boy at the bar, only that you'll have to use sign language. His lip reading isn't so fast, besides he is used to the company that does sign language like his peers at school. At home, we have videos on how to sign language, and we go to church that does sign language. He has a tutor that was also hard of hearing, and they sign language more than lip read. A cousin bought a book for sign language just to try.

Jimmy goes to the mall regularly. Janey would go to the mall often, but Jimmy was like the cool kid—he goes on the weekend when school is out. His classmates do, too. They often hung out. Jimmy would mostly be with Michelle. They've been going out since Jimmy was in junior year. Sometimes, Janey can sense Jimmy was lonely when Michelle goes out of town with her family so she'd sometimes hang out with Jimmy in the malls. Janey knows sign language, not too fast though and not as much, but she can explain herself. A funny incident happened: Jimmy was supposed to pick up prints, and Janey came along. As Janey was about to speak to the salesperson, the salesperson immediately looked down opened the drawers and looked for the prints. This confused Janey, and she asked, "You know what we're looking for?" while handing the receipt or stub. The salesperson's jaw dropped. She said, "You can speak?!" Janey smiled.

This happened on the bus, too. While riding Jimmy and Janey communicate through sign language and many stare, but when Janey requests to get off everyone is mostly wide-eyed. One cannot blame them. They've been watching Janey and Jimmy use sign language, and then speak to get off the bus all of a sudden.

Jimmy loves movies. This perplexed Janey's partner, Gayle. Janey told Gayle that they should watch a certain movie because her brother said it was awesome. Not for anything, Gayle asked which brother suggested the movie. Janey said Jimmy. Gayle asked Janey how he said so, and Janey showed her Jimmy's sign language. Imitating it so Gayle could understand. Jimmy signed: It was beautiful. The title he spelled using the sign language alphabet and it was action packed.

Beautiful in sign language is like your right palm facing your face making a circle or jellyfish like motion. Action packed is Jimmy mimicking actions of people on the movie, especially the hero.

When Janey was reviewing for her board exams which was much because she was done with school, she promised—no, she was determined— and told herself she'd get to know Jimmy even better. Janey's sign language skills improved so much when she spent an hour or two talking to Jimmy in sign. She often lurked in his bat cave those days because she had time.

Gayle loved Janey's brother. She would imitate him sometimes. She knew a little bit of sign—like tired. I'm tired or I'm puffed. She knows cute, beautiful—the basics like mom and dad. Females were below the nose, whilst male like dad, uncle, and grandpa used gestures above the nose.

I hope no one argues men are above and women below—it is just word formation. What's important is to communicate, and understand or get the message across.

Chapter 6

College and Mainstream

At a disadvantage.

Jimmy and his friends Mario, Charlie, Reese, and Lesly were all eager to go to university or college. They, like fresh, young graduates, were looking forward to solidifying their dreams, their lives.

Charlie, the second honors in their batch, went to UB. He hadn't fully cross-dressed then, but as he got older, he ultimately did—even made a name for herself on some local projects that promote LGBT. Charlie wanted to pursue Fine Arts, but even the most prestigious school in our city was not equipped for these at that time. He enquired at San Seladin University, and it was the same.

Jimmy was also filing all sorts of stuff—it was just all college application. Janey studied in not just a prestigious school known for people with high marks but where popular kids go to. Jimmy told Janey in sign language that since the university doesn't yet have a program that supports individuals with hearing disability, he will study somewhere else and transfer, hopefully, the following semester or school year. Jimmy wanted San Seladin like Janey. It was also one of the first schools Charlie applied in. Samantha, their mom, was a magna cum laude at the university. Samantha took up biology as a preparatory for medicine. Janey took up finance. So, Jimmy's batch was scattered applying to different colleges. Jimmy wanted computer or information technology.

Not to be a dark cloud, but Janey wanted to give Jimmy a piece of her mind—not to pull down his dreams or anything but Janey wanted open communication between Jimmy and herself. Janey said, remembering the time Jimmy had a tutor who was also hard of hearing, "Well," she gently asked at first, "Jimmy, why do you want to study computer technology?" Maybe, Jimmy did see this was the wave of the future so did Janey.

Janey just felt so many took up computer and ended up unemployed. The market competition for this was very stiff then, unlike at present where employment demand is now so high that it evened out the playing field for computer or information technology. Janey just shared her thoughts. She lingered as he could also be a teacher for someone like him—no one can take that away and can be his mentor or model and of course, logically, one with hearing disability can prefer someone who went through the same thing. Just Janey's thoughts.

Jimmy prepared so hard for his college application, especially the entrance exams. Samantha helped Jimmy review and study. The entrance test on one school, just at the back of our building, was computer based. Right there and then, you would know for the competency if you're a pass or a fail. To add more intensity, it was also right minus wrong.

Hurray! Our Jimmy passed! It was a celebration. Janey and her family were just so happy that the hardwork paid off. Dameon, someone from his batch, applied in the same school and he, too, passed. Hurray for mainstreaming!

After high school, these adolescents were assumed to be equipped for mainstreaming. That means they can be integrated to the normal curricula with accommodations that meet their needs. That was the thrust of the special school once graduated.

Jimmy's semester had been paid. Jimmy was all set in his new-school-new-life phase. First day, he was okay, maybe a little beat but okay.

Second day, his shoulders were slouched. He went directly to his room and did not want to explain how the day went.

This time, it was required that he wears his hearing aid or at least most of the time he had. He disliked that. He had one since he was a toddler, and his family was fearful he'd just break it since he kept pulling it off his ears.

Janey learned from Jimmy, who was older now, that he found other sounds loud and distracting. When they used sign language, it was mainly conversation and facial expressions and gestures. But he explains the door, the TV set—everything made a sound, sometimes they were loud—he had to learn to filter these sounds as those of us who hear normally disregard these things.

On the third day, he sat down and talked to the family. He would like to study in the same college as his high school friends. He learned there was somewhat a sign language translation in every class.

He said he could not make out what those beside him uttered, for example, the pencil, some people called it *lapis,* number 2 or other names, labels and terms. All these were new to Jimmy. All these were confusing, more confusing than the courses themselves. Terminologies.

In high school, it was mostly English, and he struggled all the more nowadays with the dialects or different names and labels of things, plus slang.

Jimmy was on the verge of tears.

So, just like they had not graduated as they were good friends, most of his batch in high school met again at CBU. Dameon, however, did not have problems in that new school. He finished and graduated college in that university that Jimmy left. There is a likelihood of different factors; however, Dameon pursued. That is a feather in the cap of their high school for hard of hearing: He was fully integrated and mainstreamed.

Janey's afterthought was that Jimmy was also one of the cool kids in high school, and it needed an extension. He was much closer to his batch, compared to Dameon at least. Nonetheless, everyone in the family supported Jimmy—new hearing aid and all. Also, even if in the previous school the whole school year was paid off he transferred.

Jimmy ran into a similar problem when he opened a convenience store. It was like a stall but bigger—much bigger and more products were sold. It was on the ground floor of the building. Like a stall, Jimmy was inside and buyers ideally say what they wanted to buy. When customers would ask him for food flavoring, *betsin* or *vetcin,* they mean just one thing: MSG. Originally his plan of action was having like a little piece of paper and customers scribbled what they needed to purchase, but then people were calling the same things different names like when he was in college, in the previous university. So, pointing, picking up and carrying items worked best than the pieces of paper. Different names for the same things though confused Jimmy at first, but he eventually got the hang of it when he had his convenience store.

Unlike the approach to hearing disability in the past, nowadays, early on an ear operation as a toddler is strongly encouraged and to mainstream with a special education teacher and if the need requires a teacher aid with expectations set on the onset for parent commitment. The education curriculum must be reinforced by the parent in the home—they work alongside and more immediate.

Samantha's bestfriend's daughter, Princess, had her operation early on and started mainstream at a montessori school since she started schooling. She had been equipped in this approach. Sign language is a dying breed, you could say. Rather than some trying to popularize or encourage more integration of it, ideally, lip reading or even mainstreaming after an ear operation is what is suggested. Inclusion and integration at an early age.

Janey while studying took a part time job tutoring English. She had a Korean student who knew sign language who called it hand language. They also have colloquial terms and gestures. It's not all straight up. One sign for each or universal. However, just like language is to convey ultimately there is meeting of minds in the effort of trying to understand. Other times you got to spell out what you're saying. In their culture that time, to reach out by incorporating or integrating sign language was, but that is no longer the case.

The deaf-mute, hearing-impaired, hard of hearing community on the outside looking in is very close knit. They have people from abroad all the time. They show them around. Being smaller in number has made them closer and more accommodating.

In Jimmy and Janey's building, they had a chef from Hawaii who was hard of hearing. He usually stayed half a year. For about two years, he did so.

Interjecting hothead…

It cannot be helped for men to run into a fight. Khalid, the chef who rented, on one occasion bought beer from Jimmy's convenience. Jimmy just plastered a signage of an increase in prices of the beverages; however, Jimmy's dad, Matthew, who wanted to lend a hand at the store did not read the new price posted. He sold Khalid the usual. Khalid came back after a while to buy more drinks. And this time, Jimmy was at the store, and Khalid was surprised in the price difference. *He thought it was to get more money out of him.* He didn't budge yet. The group got to drinking. It was almost close to Khalid leaving again, so he wanted to treat his friends to a few more rounds. Jimmy joined in, and in one of their conversations, Khalid, intoxicated with alcohol, blurted out why he was charged different amounts for the beer on the same day. Jimmy tried explaining. Unexpectedly, they got into a fist fight. Matthew, worried, instructed Janey to call the police. Janey thought hard, protective of her brother. They were nearby a station though and, by some coincidence, the SWAT, not the normal police, passed by. The SWAT halted the fight. They were supposed to bring Khalid to the station just so he can cool off they said. Janey was so amazed at the girlfriends of her brother and Khalid's during this incident. It was in the nick of time Jimmy got in the building in the middle of the fight because Michelle came down, snapped at Jimmy. Jimmy even pretended to lie on the ground, which scared Matthew when he saw his son lying down, but Janey knew he was just being drunk and pretending because Michelle slapped him and called him out to stop, and they went in the building to their floor. The SWAT arrived a few seconds, and Khalid was still fuming. Another girl impressed me—Jessica, Khalid's girlfriend, came between Khalid and the SWAT who was about to take Khalid away. She was also hard of hearing and couldn't explain herself explicitly. With tears streaming down her face, she pleaded for the SWAT to not take Khalid away. Janey interceded. They were throwing a going-away party, Janey explained that Khalid is leaving, and it got a little heated, but it is okay now that everything has been explained. The SWAT issued a warning and gave way.

It was the first time Janey saw a gold customized .45 owned by one of the SWAT. A golden pistol doesn't come along daily.

Janey reckons how girlfriends and partners can essentially put you in your place.

Khalid and Jessica are especially naughty and kinky as a couple. Janey recalls passing by their room hearing tasers. There would be electric bleeps. They taze each other. Janey's unsure either their walls to the room are too thin but you could overhear them in the bathroom fiesty there too. * smirk

A few days later, Khalid left. He left a long apology letter to the family. He mentioned he had issues with the WIFI but never complained. Janey winced knowing she turns the WIFI off when she arrives after getting off from work. Rumor also came about Khalid wanting to buy the old building then, and Sam, Jimmy and Janey's youngest brother, retorted, **"He even complained about the price of beer, and he wants to buy our building."** That was some incident. The long apology letter was moving though and Khalid extended respects in the midst.

That was some male beef.

Peering Through the Keyhole is also about a spot on the planet—the space, place, and time element. It is about the challenges, heartwarming, clenching, riveting events close to ground zero of hearing disability, such as withstanding the hothead incident. A viewpoint heavily impacted by these events with hands tied, like whether they wanted to or not, they just are.

Flashback: Prior encounters with the authorities
Two marked incidents

Janey could not help but think Jimmy looked extremely goodlooking that day. A yellow T-shirt made him somewhat a little tan. Tan isn't so brown but has a hint of blush or pink, not pale. He had his gel, his deep eyes, and dark brows.

He and Michelle were attending a party. He wasn't driving yet. They were younger. He took a cab to Michelle's. They took a cab to the party and taking Michelle home, but he opted to commute on his way home himself. At the corner where Michelle lived, some bystanders asked him money out of the blue which stunned the young boy. They took out knives and got his money. Arriving home, he was so frustrated. They reported everything to the police. They had to go to the station near Michelle's to identify the individuals. He vented out, "Why would they ask me money? I don't know them. I don't owe them."

He had not worn that flashy T-shirt for some time. He feels he attracted unwanted attention.

One time, on his way home from public commute on the bus, the house well, building shook with a scream the moment he got home. He was holding it in. Someone sat beside him, pulled out a revolver and asked for his money again.

This was the second time—thank goodness the last time! But Jimmy…he gave his money, his allowance. He was very good at budgeting and saving. He screamed so loud and he wanted to buy his own gun for a while.

Incidents in the past. Times are better now. Unfortunately, there can be added safety in one's own vehicle.

Janey had her fair share of incidents. It's unlike Jimmy's though. The milder one was when she traveled with her Auntie Ginnie and cousin to Siargao. When she got back, her room was broken into, because she had her own floor. She reported that to the police.

Janey, when younger, she also wore flashy clothes. I don't know if it screams steal-from-me. But she was from a building on another block. It was their cousin's, that building. She stole some pictures coming from other cousins who had spent a vacation with them so she could have copies herself. She thought it was karma. This was their modus. People had heard this on the news. She wore blue. It was her favorite. She looked good in blue, and white denim jeans. However, her wallet was showing on her back pocket. It wasn't small that could be kept fully in the pocket. That was when it happened. The MO—the modus. She walked facing a man whose eyes were very red; she almost thought, in prejudice, he took drugs. She felt relieved when they were passed each other; however, the man, after they had passed, backed up a little bit and pulled her protruding wallet from the back pocket. She worried if he could be bringing anything—a knife or something sharp of that kind. When she turned around, the man hurried on a back of a motorcycle. She was not pursuing that, but she managed to scream "Thief! Thief!" loudly, and the man fell off the motorcycle before getting back on again. That was the funnier thing. He fell off. Too bad they managed to take her wallet.

Janey had an incident in her college, along the campus at around 6 P.M. She wasn't feeling very well. Someone got off the bus and pulled her hand. He seemed to have wanted her cellphone, but if he'd pulled that he would have gotten it. Mistakenly, he pulled her arm. And they did a tug of war a little bit on the street. Janey was with Gayle then who was so wide-eyed on what to do. Janey thought of picking up something to hit the guy's head with but he immediately got on the bus after the little tug of war. She learned this was another MO.

Unfortunately, no, luckily, there were no knives or guns. Thank goodness! Unlike with Jimmy, who must have been really shaken.

Chapter 7

The Work

Why don't I have work now? And I am hard of hearing?

OJT: On the Job Training, or intern.

Jimmy and his batch in college were busy looking for work, so they can complete the necessary hours as a requirement for school prior to graduation.

Some companies also have a program where they hire individuals with special needs, specifically, as a community outreach.

While some of his batch approached these organizations, others had family whose business they can work for.

Janey was so eager about the news of Jimmy "working". She couldn't keep her mouth shut. She blurted out to Samantha. Samantha from teaching medical students or interns now work with the government. Ordinarily, they hire encoders, since Jimmy took up computers as he wanted, he could very well meet the requirement as an encoder for starters or for the time being. The pay is better in the government. However, what might not have been clear in the beginning was this was only on a job-order basis, and Samantha was very eager to work with her son. Most job orders, renew and continue anyway.

Jimmy was so eager to work. He would sometimes leave and go in earlier than Samantha. The job order was under Samantha's.

In all honesty, Samantha found it challenging to instruct things. Maybe some special needs training were crucial, but she was his mother. She knew the basics to sign language, and she had a bit of competency in teaching yet she admitted it was challenging.

Janey, on the other hand, admired Jimmy's work ethics. Although, Samantha never came to work late, but Jimmy, maybe because work was new to him, tirelessly went with their mom or even ahead of her to the office. They also did a lot of long hours to compensate for more delays on the encoding process because of the challenges. Some instructions were hard to convey; hiccups need to be ironed out but, coming home late and leaving the house early, Jimmy kept going. And, his spirits were always up.

Until, they met a fork in the road. Jimmy was luckier the government's pay is better than the rest of his peers. Some became regularized though or permanent, absorbed by the company, while Jimmy's job order ended in six months. The school only needed three months, so he was working the rest of the months, but it ended.

Jimmy's questions about why he doesn't have work and being hard of hearing crushed Janey's heart. Janey was informed that it was because the project was over. It was hard to make Jimmy understand.

Samantha felt her heart was pierced. She thought if she had not insisted to help or wanted to work alongside Jimmy, things might be different. Janey felt guilty, too, if she had not been so eager to spill about Jimmy needing to intern, and they just let Jimmy be maybe he could have found another internship and be permanent or absorbed in companies like his friends.

The first couple of months he was working, Jimmy bought his digital camera. It wasn't surprising Jimmy liked things—specific things, nice things, and durable things. He had good taste. Sometimes, Janey just liked pretty, shiny things. What Janey liked to do was take her family out. There was always that…a date—a date with all of them, a date with Matthew, a date with Samantha, a date with Jimmy, and a date with Sammy, their youngest. Or with the whole bunch, why not?

It took some time for Jimmy to bounce back. The family usually saw Jimmy hang out with his friends in his room. He had a larger room in the building. Samantha, one time, ran into Reese, Jimmy's ex and also batch while many of them were hanging out in Jimmy's room. "Why are you all here?" Samantha asked with a smile. Samantha kind of had an idea. Reese replied, "Because we don't have work. We are jobless."

Although some of them were fortunate on landing on a job, a number weren't.

After awhile Jimmy started his convenience store. He also managed some rooms for rent on the building.

But eventually, he got into a 9-to-5.

In the middle of all this, he also got back to school and took up teaching or Special Education (SpEd) like Janey wanted for him. He was influenced by Michelle, his girlfriend and live-in partner.

Remember him waiting for her and picking her up every day at school. She took up teaching, SpEd at that. Jimmy got rallied by people or a change of heart that he re-enrolled taking the same, and so he has two majors, the first, computer technology, and a degree in Special Education.

Chapter 8

A Talk

Remain composed.

Jimmy and Janey are older now. Both working. Nah, it was Jimmy at this time while Janey was reviewing for her board exams in finance.

Jimmy approached his older sister who was seated on the sofa in the dining area near the kitchen.

"Janey," he asked, "Why aren't you married yet? Why don't you settle down?"

Jimmy then added, "Are you worried about me? I can handle myself."

Although Janey felt her head spin suddenly. She was dizzy, but she knew, before the questions, that she felt great. *It was an ordinary day gone awry.*

Janey swallowed hard, but she wasn't letting her cool or composure slip. Saying, *Keep it together* in silence. She said, "Of course not." Although she does. Taking care of Jimmy, she feels, crosses every family member's thoughts once or twice. An aunt even wanted to adopt him! But it's not only the thing we think about, not even always. But it's like we have an unspoken promise to do our best.

Janey always repeats to herself that essential restraint to give him leg room to grow. He could even turn out better than Janey, or whatnot. The future is unwritten and to be made. The situation only counts 10% while reaction 90% people say.

You are not your circumstance. You can change that. Do your best to.

Essential restraint. Janey practiced that ever since they were children, at a distance looking out for Jimmy. He'll be able to manage himself. He may need a hand, a nudge every now and then like all the rest of us. But he'll manage like he did when he made friends and traded his cards. Life.

Chapter 9

Everyone's Living Arrangements

This was when Janey started to lose Jimmy.

"A wedge has been thrust between us."

Janey and Jimmy's parents left for Australia with Sam for good, leaving Janey in charge of the household while they tried settling in. They had turned the building from accepting tenants to a regular family home. There may be somebody else living with them but unlike before where it was a business that they were known for. Every once in a while, they had someone or a couple or two who needed a place to stay for short term, unlike before they could have twenty to thirty tenants. Now it was just down to one or two, at the most four. It was such waste of space. Few tenants had been the arrangement for a decade now. Samantha and Matthew hadn't given up their jobs yet, but they were very near retirement. Sammy just finished nursing. Their family in Australia was huge, so it's going to be a great opportunity. They will be living in their own place, twenty minutes from the ocean. It is going to be a lot of fresher air and sea breeze.

Jimmy and Janey's grandparents have passed, so it seems they practically own the building. It was even hard to figure if the school would continue to run and who'll stay in the house by the coast. Good thing! Before Jonathan's passing, Benjamin, Samantha's brother took on helping by the coast, and so it was normal or convenient transition for Benjamin to continue running the school. He also had the degree. While Samantha's household ran the building for rent since they had been there for ages. It was assumed for convenience in arrangement that Benjamin and Samantha who have settled in their roles just continue in their respective roles.

A bit of ruckus started after Janey, too, left for the Middle East, undecided whether for vacation or for good.

Janey manned the little household smoothly. She had work as a teacher. She took teaching or education as a second degree course after finance. While Jimmy attended to his convenience store. Michelle, Jimmy's girlfriend, continued to live with him since the college she was studying in was within walking distance. Normally, before she would head home, she would hang around the building, or if she had a long vacant period at school, she'd drop in too. But they, and I think, she, too, got used to hanging around Jimmy and her sleepovers, she did not get along with her brother. Whilst Michelle was very welcome in their home. Sammy, before Australia, had a girlfriend living with Janey and Jimmy. She was really from out of town and instead of having to pay rent to attend college in the city where she met Sammy, she lived with them, too. She could visit her siblings, who rented around the city. She almost seemed like a tenant, but she stayed for free. Sadly, she and Sammy weren't able to withstand an LDR or long distance relationship.

Samantha and Matthew would be home every once in a while, since she was just consuming her leaves and retiring so was Matthew.

The time zone and the jetlag blew their minds. They'd wake up at dawn and strike a conversation if you go out for water in the kitchen. Someone would be wide awake when you pass by the living room, or they would instead sleep in so late in the day. It was awake at dawn wanting to talk or sleeping in the day like a vampire. That was jetlag.

When work arrangements were done, they left portions of their pension to Janey for the building, as they also found work in Australia anyway. Although retired, a few more years didn't matter. They thought. To keep them busy day to day in Australia.

Janey assumed the role to a tee. She ran the building like a ship or clockwork. She always waited for Jimmy for the weekend groceries they do. She plotted their meals for the week. They would often go out—Janey, Jimmy, and Michelle—as soon as the pensions were out. Janey hated having to go pay the bills then, unlike now where everything is done online. The lining up was such a waste of time.

At first, it didn't feel so much like they were moving to a different country until it finally sank in.

Life in a new city is absolutely not easy. Sammy had to leave Dianne, his girlfriend, whom he met in nursing. They ultimately could not handle the distance and broke up. Sammy met Veronica, not a coworker, but also a nurse. It took some time for another steady relationship. They've been together for a while. Their relationship can be a bit perilous like two difficult people not really peas of a pod.

When everything in Australia settled in, Samantha worked as a medical coder manager, whilst Matthew was a caregiver. Sammy soon found work as a nurse. At first, he was a cashier, a job he landed on while he was prepped for the requirements to be a nurse. They agreed that for Matthew, as he was getting a lot older and his caregiver's job involved a lot of manual labor, it was best he took care of the things around their apartment, mostly just cooking. Their finances could manage. Matthew attended to picking up Samantha from work. He would sometimes hang around other seniors, meaning senior citizens, at the home he passed by, grab a cup of milk, coffee, and a little meal before heading to Samantha's office.

Whilst Janey thought she was running a tight ship. They had a houseboy who helped around the cooking and cleaning of the building, Jimmy attended to his convenience store. His beverages were booming, especially the alky; however, his hours were long around lunch. He used a louder buzzer, so he doesn't miss a customer. Even their room, his and Michelle's, had a light instead of a buzzer as a doorbell, which serves more effective to call their attention since they're both hard of hearing. They rely heavily on their vision, compensating. However, loud sounds also do the trick in catching their attention.

Janey decided to visit Gayle who moved to the Middle East. They have kept toe-to-toe and Janine, Gayle's partner, and her were good friends. Janey even thought to work or move to the Middle East for the experience, but she wasn't fully committed. Her going was to get the feel. Janey went to the Middle East for a month which turned to two months since Gayle wanted her to stay longer. She extended but her visa was just up to that.

Janey had a wonderful experience. She was about to work. But she wanted to forego the working opportunity since work back home wasn't that bad, she reckons. She also made arrangements in case she'd go back. Although, she was about ready to work there en route to Australia to her family. She had even given things away. She came home though but wanted to keep visiting Gayle and Janine. As a couple, they've been together almost two decades. They broke up in the middle. Gayle had short term partners in between. Surprisingly though, even if they were engaged, they broke up permanently. They've bought a condo together but have officially broken up and broken off the engagement.

The building and pensions were left with Jimmy. When home, Janey was supposed to handle everything again from the building and household to the bills. Janey, however, mentioned her frustrations, such as lining up for payments of the utilities not being set up online yet at that point, to Samantha. Jimmy having Persons-with-Disability (PWD) benefits had a special queue in every place so it was definitely easier for him. They had privileges, you see, even in parking vehicles. Jimmy was also more comfortable paying the bills. It did not pose such headache, unlike for Janey.

While Janey was away, Jimmy closed his convenience store. They had a few tenants, and he added more. Coincidentally, some of Michelle's siblings were remodelling their own houses and needed a place to stay while they were being built or construction work was completing. Jimmy realized the pensions and rent brought more money than working in the convenience store, spending long hours tending the store, including slow hours, example, certain times during the day where there are less customers. Tedious.

Janey liked the idea Jimmy handled some of the bills, she had not thought her coming home, although Jimmy was pleased to see her, would jeopardize their relationship. Jimmy started charging her for more electricity and other bills. The other tenants said the same. Jimmy was stingy with money. Of six tenants, Samantha left one for Janey so she'd receive rent from one, but Jimmy took over all the apartment rent, thinking it was only left to him. In the past, Janey had her friends crash or live at the building for a while, and she received a little rent. They could both have rent, you see. Janey had access to her coworkers, while Jimmy and Michelle had Michelle's siblings and a few others. Jimmy took this sourly or with a lot of distaste. Janey, it seems, had a lot when she came home, and it felt different.

Chapter 10

A Marriage

No.

Janey's brother living with his partner for years wanted their parents blessing to get married since they are of age, and it was more triggered by Michelle's sister wanting to marry. In our culture, ideally, the elder sister should marry ahead of the younger one if they were both in long term relationships. It's like respect. Not all, but being the older sibling you, most likely or more often than not, you might miss the opportunity to marry. You get teased, in most instances, even if they keep rallying that we each have our own clock and pace.

Jimmy had been living with Michelle for years. I don't know if it's the circumstance. Why pop the question now? Was it the had-to factor or that Samantha and Matthew said no? It wasn't because of both of them being hard of hearing. It was more because of the pending processing of immigration papers.

Jimmy and Michelle had been together since Jimmy was in junior year in high school. Jimmy became a grade or year level higher than Michelle because, even if Jimmy stopped school due to his car accident, Michelle quit school some time ago to spend time traveling with family. Thank the stars they met in school. Although by coincidence, they had this cute picture together when they were in grade school. They hadn't known each other then. It was a random picture that surprised them. Wow! They had already met back then. They were three in the photo. It was with a common friend to both, and this photo had been framed in Jimmy's room for the longest time since he was in grade school. So, their relationship can be glorified or destined, quote unquote, by this incident or photo. They used to sign language "quite odd and absurd" referring to the whole thing. They were three. They looked so happy, great smiles, but the one in the middle knew them, not them! Jimmy also always found it odd that on Janey's baby book she was named Michelle, but they changed it to Janey. Jimmy figured this out himself like when Janey when he had nothing better to do and would go over old things around the house, including this baby book. Janey found out and mentioned it to their parents afterwards. Unknowingly, the baby book was left lying around, and Jimmy took a look. Then he made a joke and laughed about it much then. Jimmy used to tease Janey that she was adopted because why'd she have a different name, and by perfect coincidence, his older sister has the same name as his girlfriend, Michelle.

As live-in partners, it hasn't been smooth sailing between Jimmy and Michelle. They had their fair share of big fights. Jimmy, some time ago, sent a text message to Samantha, which she kept on her cellphone, saying: PLEASE HELP ME FIND THE WORDS. I CAN'T EXPLAIN TO MICHELLE HOW I FEEL. That shot to the core—even people who can utter or talk have difficulty expressing themselves sometimes, how much harder was it that Jimmy was feeling?

A large part of communication is typically learned unconsciously through hearing something and imitating even the basic sounds and phonetics.

Admittedly or almost always, other senses compensate. That is always the case; however, what some may take for granted on a daily, some struggle harder with inadequacy.

Janey witnessed how Jimmy loved Michelle since they were younger when they hung out at the mall with friends, and Jimmy used to put his hand in Michelle's denim pants back pocket, so it's like he'd go wherever Michelle went. He'd be tagged along, trudging on the pants. Janey hung out with Jimmy, and Janey would learn that Michelle was traveling with family because Jimmy would explain missing Michelle. He'd sometimes even put his hand in Janey's back pocket instead, saying that's what he usually does to Michelle at the mall. Jimmy would re-enact it whenever he misses Michelle. Janey would smile.

To when they had a big fight and Michelle moved out for a while. Some other guy picked her up, and Jimmy dated another girl. As Matthew was surprised to see another girl, he said, with Jimmy, Janey expected it was going to be quite a challenge no one knew each other for so long or had been together for so long. What irked Janey was when Jimmy, because there is social media now, wrote: Yes, I miss you. I miss f—ing you. Clearly, not an adult yet then, but they've moved passed that.

Jimmy adored Michelle. Janey never saw her brother clean any room before Michelle officially moved in and most absolutely not his, and how he did the laundry and cooked. At first Janey and her parents thought Michelle was going to be living a life of a princess.

Before Michelle moved in, while in Jimmy's room, they would run in Michelle sleeping cozily on the bed while Jimmy was on his couch.

Jimmy and Michelle have been through many routines over time: from Jimmy first going to college and them rarely seeing each other to Michelle being a grade or year level lower in high school. They would have a meeting place at the end of the day. One time, Jimmy's cellphone, which Matthew bought that he asked for, was stolen from Michelle's backpack while she was on the way to meet Jimmy. Jimmy was so frustrated and worried how to tell Matthew. He lost another one of Matthew's given phones—all these phones were his choices—in a cab. It's hard. He goes by vibration; he, as well as Michelle, cannot really notice if it falls off due to their ***hearing disability.***

When Jimmy was working at the encoding job, he had to do overtime to get a hang of the job. You could really sense on Jimmy's face that he could not wait for the weekend. Absolutely, he'd meet Michelle.

And when Michelle moved in while she was taking up a teaching course for special education at the university near where they lived, Jimmy would pick her up daily.

It's a romance with routines and has coped over time.

Some worst times were when Jimmy was in a bender. It started that he was upset with something else. Sometimes, he drinks a bit too, and he would vent his frustrations that he was out of work. How can he then support a family, if ever? He is prudent and cautious to think about these. But it got somewhat better when he got back to school taking up the course Janey wanted, which was perfect or a mere coincidence again because he followed Michelle instead of just picking her up every day. He, eventually, enrolled, too. Happily, he was amazed most students at that university knew sign language; they had a platform for it. Unlike when he was mainstreamed or finishing his computer course at that other university or college, they practically had an interpreter at every class. In Michelle's university, he could communicate with more people.

The cause of the bender: He would lash out a bit even cry like in frustration about the opportunities of the future and having a family.

Janey once asked Michelle, this was years since they have been together, "Do you love my brother?" Her response was, "Before, I'm sure I used to. Now, I'm not sure." They talked in sign language. Janey laughed, amused. She thought, *Michelle was too honest. Maybe she forgot that I'm his sister.* ☺

Eerie interlude…

An incident on a March, roughly three months from Michelle's mother passing, Janey came home to a wailing. Someone crying heavily as she neared the living room. It was Michelle. She thought at some point that it was her breaking point. She saw Michelle to be very tough, but she also saw how close she was to her mom, so she knew at some point Michelle would break. A friend and tenant before too had his dad passed, and, sometimes at night when Janey came down, she'd hear that tenant sobbing for weeks. Michelle had a few drinks because Jimmy drank some alcohol. Jimmy was on a videocall with their parents in Australia he offered his sister a drink. Janey said no. Jimmy retorted, "You're trying to be a do-gooder in front of the camera or videocall." It wasn't that. Janey thought, *What else would happen if everyone were drunk.* Michelle was already sobbing, and Jimmy almost lost it and fell while he was fetching something from the little pantry. Janey had a good sense to call their Uncle Vinny who can maneuver easily to the building with his motorbike. He picked Jimmy up who fell at the dry pantry. He settled him on like a camping blanket near there to rest, while Michelle was already on the couch, Janey just unfolded a sofabed and decided to call it a night, watching over them, and their Uncle Vinny left after settling Jimmy. Around three in the morning, Jimmy almost soundly sleeping, Janey had a sofabed to herself, and on the couch, Michelle who had long hair that reached her waist, suddenly woke up and rocked herself, just rocked. She lost her eyeballs, too, like she was possessed for a bit. Immediately, Janey called for Roberto, their houseboy who was like a working student. They were both stunned by what happened to Michelle. She got out of it though. It stopped somehow. But weirdly, the following day, she was picked up by her uncle or family, she stayed with them for a month or two before coming back to the building and she cut her hair from the waist to shoulder length. That was eerie.

She lost her eyeballs and rocked in the middle of the night; her waist length hair adding to the situation. It was good she took some time away. Maybe everything was sinking in or she was confronted by what had happened. They are twelve siblings in all, you see, and they lost both their parents to cancer. Both parents were CPAs or certified public accountants. It's not that that matters, but definitely them being orphans. They are very tight. Real close. Michelle can make clothes. She sews and does a little bit of designing as well, so whenever they have occasions, they'd all dress up in different styles but ideally using the same fabric. They always had themes. They kept themselves so close and happy even if their parents passed. It's a lovely thing.

Chapter 11

It's a Boy, a Son and His Gadgets

In the back of my mind, I don't know if we'll stay that close like we used to. I think we've lived it because ours with my sibling—it's never coming back now. We got our memories though. We're like hoping for God's miracle now.

-Janey

Jimmy and Michelle, hands down, are very smart and practical. They are quite the couple, although a couple outside of marriage, since they were advised not to wed yet. The couple managed to have a baby, a boy. It happened not when they were teens neither was it not unplanned. It happened after they were refused to wed, despite being of age.

Janey was elated. She was one of the happiest for them. She always hoped and prayed that everything would work out. Janey wanted them to even marry and almost argued with Samantha and Matthew about why Jimmy and Michelle could not. Unfortunately, that was that.

Michelle, not getting any younger, was pretty smart to conceive a boy and, *boy! was she bloated*—too bloated and fat during her gestation or pregnancy. She was under strict orders to have complete bed rest due to her age factor. Nick of time. Let this sink in for body clock. Our dreams may always be there, but time is important. Those really lucky ones.

She was a good example to her siblings. You see, the younger one ultimately married, but she had three miscarriages that almost made her lose faith and left her depressed but Michelle, the older sister that she is, had Jasper. That should challenge you.

Janey personally felt Jasper pumped blood back into Jimmy and Michelle's relationship. Remember when Michelle answered she *used to love Jimmy*? Jasper reignited this. Jasper would always look for both parents not just one, especially if his dad and *nanay* (local term for mother) were not around. He holds each one of them with each hand; he is like their eyes or ears for that matter. He'd play with his *nanay* like friends, such a lovely sight with a lot of laughter. He learned sign language on his own pretty fast, quicker than the vernacular, quicker than speaking English, because his parents are very hands on. One time, Janey and the rest were worried he'd use sign language more than his vocal chords.

Janey was one of those who pushed for Jasper to go to school, which Jimmy would later agree to. Jasper did sign language more, although he doesn't have a hearing disability. He needed exposure with kids his age. He *can* learn sign language; he can be there for his parents, but he should also be with peers his age, mostly it was his cousins at first. He almost had a global delay, especially in speech. School and tutors helped. He is doing pretty well now and still is always around his parents.

Janey would like to imagine he would someday champion them and their situation.

He had a speech therapist and a tutor for classes in school.

When Jasper was a boy, and Grandpa Matthew was visiting from Australia, while having dinner at the marina, Jasper uttered, "Sheep" while Janey was carrying him. Janey looked for what looked like a goat but Jasper pointed to the boat. He meant ship. And at a mall, he said, "Parking lot." Janey realized, as what Michelle's sisters did, that Japer likes vehicles and knows about school buses and trains. He doesn't talk, converse, or communicate much. That's what his tutor improved. Nothing like exposure also reinforces. He is not into sentences yet, but he's into words. He has words forming his vocabulary close to cars. I guess he loves his daddy's and Janey's, his aunt's, driving. He'd be in Janey's car when they'd go on a road trip but he'd have his neck stretched out, looking out for his daddy. Compared to his peers who can easily communicate in paragraphs, Jasper, is a boy who communicates in single utterances. Jasper even prefers to sign water than to say it. Something had to be done to improve this.

The pitfalls also of internet is that he picks up undesirable words. He, a three-year-old boy, picked up the F- word. His other aunts, Michelle's sisters, noticed this, too. More adult supervision and parental control over his internet usage is much in order.

Before he had his private tutor, Samantha on a videocall from Australia was teaching Jasper or whenever she came to visit, but Jasper often cries between Samantha and Matthew, and Jimmy would shush him and their session and say the boy is beat or tired.

Janey only got to spend time with Jasper during the pandemic when they absolutely had no one to leave him with. With a teaching license, Janey could teach Jasper, but she and Jimmy were starting to clash, to not see eye-to-eye. Jasper, though, enjoyed Janey since it was always like a game, child's play, when they read a book or hung out. Janey used to bribe Jasper with ice cream, chocolates, or chips when she visited their room, and then stopped. Everyone did, even Jimmy and Michelle. When Jasper, a little boy, his blood sugar went up, and he's still a kid. Now, he is fed meat; he used to just do starch and sweets or carbs and he did not get out much until school. Thank god for school, plus speech therapy and his other tutors, for Jasper to focus on communicating. Kids of parents with special needs, even those who are hard of hearing, during their reunions speak very well, fluently. Jasper needed a nudge.

The Big Nudge!

He got over it. He is so much better now.

Kids nowadays are born with gadgets. At a very young age, they sure know how to tinker or fidget with cellphones and tablets. A two-year old can even work a cellphone better than older people. It is their generation.

Jasper, on a school day, used to be so glued to his gadgets that he played until midnight or 3 A.M. Janey supposed that he is tired at school. On the weekend, sometimes his dad calls it lights out but you could hear his playing until 5AM—very likely his parents who are unaware are sound asleep since they aren't able to notice softer sounds.

But the kid changed for the better, eventually. He followed lights out!

Chapter 12

Relationship Overcast, Social Media, and Family Fund

Interlude
Present Situation: Jimmy's Meltdown

Everyone was alarmed as Jimmy's brows were so furrowed. He had been so upset his father's pension had not gone in, and he blamed his sister. In the past, their dad asked about his pension which he left with Jimmy while their mom's went to Janey. Janey helped her dad obtain records. You see, it was only rightful to check but that upset Jimmy. He was literally tailing her dad and his sister Janey with Michelle then. Tailing Janey's car with his, seeing them go to the bank and all but that was then, and they had not done that ever again. Only time Matthew is needed is when pensioners need to update yearly to the government who also check up on them. Luckily, Matthew had savings and work elsewhere, so leaving Jimmy was the "plan in place."

Jimmy too upset had a meltdown whereby Jimmy's Uncle Vinny had to go to where he and his dad were. They were scheduled to pick up Jasper from school and then head to the bank to check as to why the pension had not gone through as normal. The banker explained it does that at times—a little earlier, a little later. Jimmy got more upset it could not be determined and that to him doesn't make sense. It was too unpredictable, and he needs it to be in on time. There was just a day or so difference or change, and this just was not workable. They even went to the lengths of having the bank records printed, going to his former school to have his professor explain how he felt and explain the bank documents, not after saying bad things to Janey blaming her for everything like she again went to the bank and tampered with everything. It was a horrible fight between the siblings. That is what they are now. Jimmy is so irked by things.

Honestly, Janey feels hopeless in these events; however, she holds on to silver linings usually brought about by Jasper. She'd go back to how, because they had no choice, they would leave Jasper to be babysat by her during the pandemic only. Another stranger. After all the ruckus or fuss over the pension, while placing the reservation, Janey clearly saw Jimmy sign to their dad that she, Janey, was part of the list to their all-you-can-eat party which was in celebration of Jasper's birthday. Jimmy brought food to school for Jasper's classmates, and the family ate all-you-can- eat. Janey prepared being left out or excluded at this party, but surprisingly, Jimmy let up this time. So, she hangs on to hope. There's just been too much bad blood over the years, mainly a decade they've both been on this earth about four. That is a quarter, and it's ugly. It's gotten ugly.

F— You

Two words that set Janey flustered on a chatbox. Before leaving for the Middle East and while she was at work, there were days Jimmy would pick her up or she would bring a car. Luckily, she lives close by but the car would still be better than the commute as it goes all the way, making it seem farther. Besides, Jimmy knows she, Janey, adores Kylie, their dog. They have three dogs. Janey and Kylie just have a connection. One time, Jimmy picked up Janey on their SUV, and Kylie was happily on the back. While Janey turned to Kylie on the back, there was some sudden movement where Kylie was abruptly turned, and Janey instead kissed the dog's butt crack. He farted, too! That incident in the SUV was hilarious. Gross but hilarious.

Over the years, Jimmy and Janey, more than siblings, were friends, unlike when they were kids when they could not understand each other. They communicated. They knew they had each other, and although some tears can be mended, some egos? No. Sensitivities cannot just like a relationship with irreconcilable differences.

It started in a chat box. Funny- there had never been chat boxes or the internet before. Nearing Janey's departure for the Middle East and Samantha surprisingly came home to see her off but also had to attend to some affairs that needed to be settled. Janey was her designated driver then. Janey's friends, or a number of them took time to see her off, too. But it was clear, either for a while or just a vacation, the family's move, as a group, is to Australia.

Apart from taking Jimmy and Michelle to every newly opened restaurant when the pensions came and from piecing the bills so it is covered—Janey was thankful for that—she had work and only her bills to attend to. Sometimes, she thinks maybe Jimmy needs more or his own share of funds to be his own, to do more of the things he liked. The building, if you think about it, *should not need funds pouring in*. It had a dispute which took two decades for a ruling in their favor. It could stand alone and generate more. Because of Janey's carefree lifestyle—frequent bar hopping with friends because she was single—this caused a misalignment on their Jimmy-and-Janey tandem. Jimmy wanting to marry and settle, while Janey was still living the "life."

Jimmy accused her of possibly squandering the funds or pensions which pierced Janey. She was making every penny worth it, and with their family's move, some loans had to be attended to and settled. She managed all that. During this time, her only confidant was Yassi who she told about the expenditures. Even when Samantha asked about the loans, Janey took offense because she felt she was doing and managing the best that she could, even though she should not take offence. All the loans were paid, and there was money left. Samantha had good reason to ask, but Janey sometimes feels the walls closing in like she was a lemon squished.

Jimmy was in the right place to ask, too. But perhaps, it was the manner or the tone that Jimmy used, which was leaning towards accusing, Janey thinks. She was working, so she had money to spare but not a lot or all of it. Jimmy then typed, *F— You*, in the chatbox. Janey was unsure if he knew what that really meant and to hurt Jimmy back, Janey wrote: I DON'T HAVE A BROTHER.

She immediately removed him from her social media, too.

How do they quarrel, you ask. Janey can sign too. But the quarrel started on the internet, with the modern chat box.

2012—that was when the rift started. Their relationship was in overcast.

Over the years, they could never get past the rift and the hard pent-up emotions that were piling, like a looming dark cloud.

Janey tried to befriend him on social media or the online platform twice, sending the request but Jimmy would not budge. He took the I-DON'T-HAVE-A-BROTHER message too literally and too seriously.

When in Boracay with her friends, Janey spilled the beans and told them that she should just have unfollowed him. Janey explained she immediately removed him remembering he wrote: I MISS YOU. I MISS F—ING YOU when he and Michelle had one of their major fights. She did not want to see anything like that on social media. Everyone is on social media nowadays. But apparently, Jimmy did not think or care to post at all. They were forever in a cold war now.

She left for the Middle East. She had a few video calls and chats with Michelle. They sent collages of Kylie. Some cousins visited the building and said Kylie was too sad. He was not eating.

The Middle East was a blast, she visited Dubai. But she could go for more trips. They had like the World Trade Financial District. Janey liked that place. Souk Madinat—it was with a body of water, but unlike Venetian, it's got a different palette. It was picturesque. It's true they had a Gold Souk—Souk meant market—Gold Souk was a block of various gold. They had all sorts like a gauntlet of gold. Their metro or trains were so new. It was very clean, and their railways not too complex…yet. They had several fountains. They have a huge aquarium at the mall with divers inside when she went. And there is a snow dome at the mall too. Their mall toilets always smelled good, so maintained and had intricate designs. On her first week in Dubai, they went to Jebel Hafeet where a lot of cars parked. It was overlooking. Nearby some would go camping, others dip their feet. There was also a hot spring at the base of Jebel Hafeet mountain. This was in Al Ain.

They went to a museum. Other places—they went jogging if it was on the mornings and would grab Indian food afterwards. They ate Greek food by the marina. Janey enjoyed Iranian kebab and biryani in a few occasions, even on the plane rides heading and coming home. It was always biryani. Janey could not forget their horizon; it was almost like two suns. Sometimes in the afternoon, the sun and moon would meet in the same sky or horizon.

She was there to visit Gayle. She found work but missed Kylie too much. She was away for about two months. Heading there, she stopped by Singapore, went around, stayed with a friend for a night, but enroute home, she had a direct flight. It was like a short immersion trip, two months.

She hadn't even seen the camels yet because Gayle wanted her to stay for longer or for a while. Good thing, she'd already seen one back home at the zoo.

She watched the fountain show nearby Burj Khalifa, spent some time along the shoreline near Burj Al Arab, and she saw the biggest aquarium in a mall located in Dubai Mall with divers in it. She had great photos and time spent with friends. She met one cousin and a friend of the family who were there at the time.

She explored Dubai from Discovery Gardens to Rashidiya, even Sharjah, JBR area or Jumeirah Beach, Diera, Bur Dubai. It was extraordinary.

Coming home though, she did not expect the looming cloud to be around them—Jimmy and her—indefinitely.

Her thoughts sometimes linger back. Of course, you are from a trip. It was memorable and spent with memorable people.

Reality from the trip, Kylie was sick and not eating. They had two visits to the vet. Janey had not thought Kylie would be so weak. Apparently, they fed rice and he was used to bones and meat and sometimes dog food, not carb but protein. Janey thinks Kylie missed her too. She thought more of Kylie than most people while she was away. Her first panic attack was she missed her dog.

She got a job when Kylie was in good health. Back to working and hanging out at bars with friends. She missed driving. Her own room was good and comfy too. Later that year, she got a smart TV, moved one of the personal computers, a small fridge and better air conditioning to her room—a better bat cave.

For a moment, when Janey got back home, Jimmy's face lit up. He and Michelle picked her up at the airport but the flight arrival was earlier than scheduled. Janey was not sure they got the short notice. One of her friends and her husband fetched her and at the house while being dropped off after eating, arrived Jimmy and Michelle from the airport. That was the only short or fleeting happy moment. She saw in Jimmy's eyes he was glad. Janey was home, and maybe Jimmy's sense of no-longer-being-*alone*-home emanated, but this sense dissipated so quickly, like the vibe was Janey should not have come back. She no longer felt welcome.

They halved the pension this time to half paying the bills. Janey gave a little well enough because they calculated her share of the electricity, but Jimmy asked for more. Janey was now like paying rent, but she was always, always out. Sleeping out. Haha. Janey just always hung around her cousins.

Janey asked around about electricity cost. Her coworkers from out of town who were renting an apartment paid as much as her, and they had refrigerators running all day. Hers was just a back-up because everyone still used the family's main refrigerator. Jimmy even had his own refrigerator for his convenience store at the lower ground floor of the building. It was the other way around. Janey wasn't using too much electricity. Jimmy was.

Janey put her foot down. Benjamin, their uncle who was managing and taking over the school, came over to add a submeter. And at the end of the month, their jaw dropped. Janey was already paying double what her bill was. She made doubly sure, you see, and checked prior bills before handing additional share. She made sure it was more, and Jimmy wanted to double it, like rent. She paid an amount exactly like rent on their own building! The nerve! The audacity to charge rent from your own sister.

The facts settled it though. Samanatha just laughed about it and shrugged it off. Samantha hadn't really seen the depth of the cold war between Jimmy and Janey yet.

Everything ensued.

Bongol.

Until everything exploded like a bomb.

Janey loved singing even though she croaked like a frog. They have a running joke about how brave Janey can be singing her heart out, getting the lyrics totally wrong aside from her croaking. She wrote that on her social media in their language: lyrics, BONGOLA NAKO. Then a little later, she had breakfast out. Jimmy stormed in her room without any business saying she called him deaf?! Janey's jaw dropped then realized her social media status. It was a lyric to a song!

He was infuriated. They almost got too physical over a small thing. She could not believe it. They were not even connected on social media any more. He is spying or someone sure is and is making up stories.

A wedge has been thrust between Jimmy and Janey.

It almost blew out of proportion and then waned again, but it was neverending now.

They lived on separate floors of the building, but he stormed in her room that day.

What must he have thought?!

Chapter 13

A Cruise, A Fire and The Present

Janey would bribe Jasper with ice cream. Jasper seems to really have a liking for Janey, but there is a hierarchy: it's always his parents first, and then whoever's face is familiar. So Janey was in. Jasper sees his aunt around. Although, he is kept mostly around his parents.

Samantha, Matthew, Aunt Zoey, and Aunt Ginnie decided to gift the family with an Asian cruise—a little bit of sunshine, tropical food and paradise plus heritage or culture. Embarkation was at Singapore. They flew in, rode a van, spent a night at a hotel, and checked in on the boat the following day. They had time to spare. They went around Gardens by the Bay which was near the marina and had lunch at a fastfood along Gardens by the Bay. Soon enough, they set sail aboard the Platija del Mar.

Along with Samantha, Matthew, Jimmy's family, including Michelle and little Jasper, plus Janey, Benjamin's wife, Aunt Julie and one of their daughters, Lainey, Aunt Zoey and Aunt Ginnie made the group of 10. That was the whole bunch. They went to Penang in Malaysia and Phuket in Thailand. They watched an ice-capade. Janey loves ice-capades. They watched one at a coliseum when she and Jimmy were younger. The aunties with Auntie Julie and Lainey enjoyed zumba. The ship had so many activities to choose from. Janey took pictures enjoying the cozy cabin accommodation of the Platija. Matthew went to the casino. With his winnings, he bought a little wooden Platija del Mar souvenir, not so little it was 21 inches by 13 inches in size. Matthew was able to leave this on display at the living room at their home, meaning the building.

They just realized…well both Jimmy and Michelle already knew the new pacifier these days was a cellphone. Otherwise, Jasper would cry if he wasn't enjoying the sites. Above all, Jasper loved water. Good thing he did not jump over the cruise ship being the child that he is. However, he cried endlessly, incessantly for the swimming pool aboard that they had to take a dip even if it was late in the day or after a day tour from a stopover in either Malaysia or Thailand. Jasper came home all wet and brimming. His smile said it all.

The family photos were marvelous. Totally one for the books. Too bad Sammy and Veronica could not make it because of work. The cruise was capped with a Captain's Night Ball. A speech and toast from the captain commenced the occasion. Everyone was formally dressed and had photos with the captain. There were pirates and paintings showcased to top the night.

The cruise ended back in Singapore where they enjoyed a day tour learning about the place—its history and culture.

Samantha loved the Botanical Gardens. This time another tour aboard a bus. They took a van from the airport to their hotel the first day, but the rest of the trip were mostly chauffeured buses of the cruise or tour packages tied up with the cruise and the tour in Singapore.

They saw the baby Merlion, the Mother Merlion because these were along the bay unlike the Daddy Merlion which was in Sentosa. Janey knew because it was her third time in Singapore. She went back for a fourth quickly, too, with a cousin and Uncle Vinny.

However, this cruise was wonderful, especially the family meals when everyone was seated together.

Sometimes it is like that. It is like it's been so long. We have our day to day lives but to come together, to make time once in a while is splendid bliss!

The family was caught up again. To each his or her own…until the fire.

It was a little over a year and a month or so from the cruise. While Janey was at work, her job was graveyard shift. She went along her day or night around her colleagues when she noticed she got several phone calls around two in the morning. She left her phone in the locker and checked in around five. She called one of the numbers, her cousin, Ivy, picked up. Janey had two phones—one, the older model, had Ivy's number but the other one, the newer model, didn't. Janey did not recognize the number right away.

"Hey you called so late." It was late in the night for regular people not doing graveyard.

"Your building caught fire," said the voice on the line. It was Ivy.

What?! Janey thought. Most calls were made at 2 A.M., and it was already 5.

Though shocked, Janey responded, "How is everyone?"

Ivy said, "Everybody's safe and okay."

Whew, Janey thought.

"Thank god," she replied. "That's such good news." Whatta relief. There is absolutely nothing we can do now. A fire and the calls were 2 A.M., it was 5.

Her coworkers overheard everything. They went ahead and told her manager who immediately said, "Go home! Now!"

What was she to expect when she got home?

There were fire trucks and lots of people on the road. She absolutely had nothing but her car and her documents. She was filing for a promotion and gathering her certificates which she conveniently puts together. These were all she has, nothing else.

No shoes other than the one she had on, a white V-neck shirt, a denim jacket she often wears when working on a graveyard shift, her pants, and her favorite black medium sized cozy bag with a sling.

What happens after a fire?

Jimmy cried over his cat, Kendal. Growing up, Jimmy had mice, hamsters, birds, a rabbit, and dogs but he seems particularly close to persian cats. Kendal had a little play area between Jimmy, Michelle and Jasper's room and their kitchen. The firefighters were not able to get Kendal, the persian cat, out of the fire.

Jimmy wanted to go back inside, but he was stopped by a firefighter. Jimmy trying to go in to save Kendal was caught on video.

A lot were lost in the fire. Janey had lost everything in the fire. Since she was at work, Janey wasn't able to save any of her belongings. Janey and Jimmy's parents had so much of their belongings left in the building. Good thing they moved and took some of their belongings with them but there were still a lot left. Some of the items lost in the fire included a collection of jewelries, housewares, such as lovely, intricately designed plates and cutlery collected over time as well as the Christmas decorations that too were collected over time. The convenience store, although closed, and Samantha's old clinic or office she used when she had patients over and other clients as she helped other doctors with epidemiology or a kind of research were also burned to the ground.

A fire is a fire.

Luckily, Jimmy, Michelle, and Jasper were on the lower ground and so several of their things were saved, especially Jimmy's car.

Janey took her car, was with her to work, so their cars were both saved.

For eleven years, their family, especially their parents, maintained Aunt Ginnie's condominium unit by the mountains. Sometimes, they go there for a dip in the swimming pool, or for some parties, they book the function areas and can easily celebrate special occasions there.

Immediately, after the fire, they were instructed to move in. Lainey was staying there at this point but mostly just on the weekends or if she's in the city. It's a two-bedroom flat with a maid's quarters and three bathrooms. Eventually, the maid's quarters was altered into a walk-in closet by everyone as it was conveniently beside one of three bathrooms. The floor area is not bad since it's a little over a hundred unlike some typical apartments, and the view is breathtaking. One could get a great view of the mountain tops down to the city with all the building lights that were mostly lit at night all the way to the ocean. It was all in sight. Surreal, visitors often say. The location, well, view gets praised a lot. The compound of the condominium unit included a gym, a tennis court, a basketball court, a swimming pool with a huge pantry nearby in case one would be cooking while enjoying swimming, and a grilling area for barbecue. It's fully equipped for unwinding and hosting a banquet and having guests over. The pantry had cutlery available for use. There was an AVR or audio-visual room, a library, and a game room with pool tables.

Jimmy felt that he lost part of his "livelihood" but he was already working in a company when the fire happened. He just thought there could be money in collecting rent from tenants.

And so, both Jimmy and Janey had work. The only problem everyone had at the condominium was parking. Since Lainey primarily stayed in the unit but wasn't there daily, she had seniority or priority over the one parking space. If she and her car weren't around, Janey could take over temporarily, but if Lainey was around, Janey would park at the visitors' parking, just like Jimmy.

Lainey shared her room with Janey, while Jimmy, Michelle and Jasper had the masters bedroom to themselves, already with a bathroom.

Lainey was assigned elsewhere for work, so she moved out. Janey missed her. She had gotten used to their weekends or whenever Lainey was around, they'd grab fastfood. Order in, stay in, lounge in, talk or be in each other's phones glued to episodes of series. Janey enjoyed having company. Jimmy had his little own family. Janey had Lainey for a while. Janey always looked forward to Lainey arriving. Eventually the parking sitch was fully sorted when Lainey moved out. Janey permanently took over while Jimmy rented a space of his own for parking within the compound. The rent, in addition to everything else, was steep, but each had their parking. Janey used most of the allotted pension for her for the payments of their new place.

The nook or new bat cave was beyond words. It was perfect, not as spacious as when Jimmy and Janey each had their own floors in the building though, and now they are sharing the same space. The old building was never with luxurious amenities like they have now. The building was built in the 1920s, the same birth year of their granddad, Jonathan, which he said he bought it because of that reason. "It is the same year as my birth, the same age as I am." Their new living arrangement was very competitive if not a cut above the rest. It's one of the sought after places in their city.

Janey could not foresee what the future holds. She and Jimmy, it seems, are forever at an impasse or disagreement. Separately, unnerved, nonchalant.

Jasper was too young to have had this roller coaster of emotions or life. Janey wondered what they'll be through his eyes—parents hard of hearing, traveling the world or the Asian cruise at a very young age, and a fire that damaged his first home.

Some may have some of these experiences, but he has it all together.

For Janey, it has spanned decades. If she plays everything through her eyes looking through a lens, it has been riddled with a lot of happy moments playing as children, family going on a cruise being the most recent, struggles—the car accident, challenges of school, work, marriage, moving, irreconcilable differences—are components or facets of a life.

This is her truth; this is her life.

Impacted and close to ground zero.

You are never alone. Whether you feel alone, want to be alone, or strive for your own, life is intertwined. You are an influence if not you make an impact on people's lives.

Think about that for a second. Be your truth. Be kind. The least you could do is not make it unbearable.

After the fire, one of Jimmy and Janey's grandparents died—Matthew's mother, Priscilla. She was near centennial—ninety-nine and six months. She was also born in 1920. They were about to be centenarians. Janey and her family were preparing for her centennial birthday. But everyone was abruptly uprooted from different parts of the world for the funeral instead of the centennial celebration.

Then the pandemic hit. She won't even get to that, but that more than rocked planet earth. The wheels perfectly oiled or changing over time changed in a matter of days or weeks. One day, you are at the office, the next you are working from home and wearing PPEs when going out. PPEs, Personal Protective Equipments. Others were working this day and no longer the following.

Scarcity and ghost town.

Janey personally quit work because she worried since she there were people who are hard of hearing with her at home. If she brings the virus, how hard it'd be for them to explain themselves in the hospital. But her employers offered her work from home.

Hopefully, we have fully made it from that peril.

And then a storm hit our city. It isn't like Janey is counting all these ominous events. Murphy's Law, when it rains, it pours—it is even more of dancing in the rain. The silver lining they say, the good side. Janey and Jimmy "somehow" have posh living arrangements. Although Janey misses the old building, she had parties there for sixty people. There are function areas in the condominium but they have to pay for the use of space; however, being in a unit, the fee is minimal in comparison to spaces this size in other party places.

Apparently, more posh need more funds. To think they used to have their own building, albeit Grandpa's. They had a basketball court too, but here is so bougie. Bling.

During the funeral, those who were undecided to come home for the centennial birthday party just showed up. It was like family you missed were instantly home. This was family on Matthew's side. The family on the cruise was from the side of Samantha.

Profoundly, Janey's city withstood that tornado too.

Janey and her family made it through the pandemic. They will sail on in this life.

At the moment, Janey caught an illness. She is going through therapy. Life, she can stare face to face, has been a celebration, not all good but also bad. Maybe one would say not all up but including the down because who says the down is not redirection to something better than what one thinks is best. Into the unknown it is, clutching what one already has or what one has been made as their tools. It is true what they said until you can say *thank you*.

Jimmy and Janey are now middle aged. Other lives maybe harsher, harder, simpler, less eventful than theirs but it's finite. If you don't live your dreams, you will work building someone else's.

A little take away, a little highlight:

"I hope you see the two suns in Dubai on one horizon. Sometimes, at a certain time of day, the sun and moon are aligned. To me, they are like two suns.

I hope you taste the smaller and sweeter buko in Thailand. World, there is so much of you.

I hope you know

Love is expressed in routines over time.

Love withstands changes.

And letting someone stand alone is the hardest part so they do well by themselves.

I was prepping for Europe before I went to therapy

We'll see how it goes.

Gotta keep a list, so we don't get sidetracked."

Janey

www.ingramcontent.com/pod-product-compliance
Ingram Content Group UK Ltd.
Pitfield, Milton Keynes, MK11 3LW, UK
UKHW040633210725
6984UKWH00014B/48

9 798896 901877